Dr. Salvatore G. Matheson

Embracing The Journey Of Vegetable Taste

Exploring The Science, Strategies, And Benefits ofi Eating And Trying New Flavors

This book was professionally typeset on Reedsy
Find out more at reedsy.com

Contents

1.

2.

3.

4.

5.

6.

7.

8.

9.

10.

11.

12.

13.

Introduction

The book of Embracing the Journey of Vegetable Taste: Exploring the Science, Strategies, and Benefits of Eating and Trying New Flavors is an enthralling investigation of how our perception of taste changes and adapts to our surroundings. Genetics, cultural backgrounds, and personal experiences all have an impact on our taste preferences. We can become more receptive to exploring new flavors and cuisines if we embrace this journey, resulting in a more diverse and delightful culinary experience. This book goes into the difficult process of taste adaptation, offering tactics and recommendations for adding salads and vegetables to your diet and, eventually, changing your taste preferences and the pleasure of these healthful foods.

Why Do People Dislike Salads And Vegetables?

Salads and vegetables may be disliked for a variety of reasons, including flavor, texture, and cooking methods. Salads and vegetables are disliked for a variety of reasons, including:

1. **Taste:** Because of the presence of plant bioactives, which are designed to defend plants from environmental stress and predators, vegetables might taste bitter. Some people may have a more sensitive bitter taste receptor, making them less inclined to enjoy salads and vegetables.

2. **Texture:** Some people find the texture of vegetables to be unpleasant. Raw veggies may have a rough or fibrous texture that makes them unpleasant to consume. Experimenting with different textures, such as slicing veggies smaller or chunkier, might aid in the discovery of a more appealing texture.

3. **Preparation:** The manner in which salads and vegetables are prepared has a significant impact on their taste and appeal. If the ingredients aren't fresh or the dressing is excessively strong, the dish will be less enjoyable to consume.

4. **Associated health advantages:** The perceived flavor or texture of vegetables can frequently overwhelm their health

benefits. Salads may be associated with diet and limitations in the minds of some people, leading to a negative opinion of the food. People are more likely to like vegetables when they are labeled with taste-focused labeling than when they are taught about their health advantages, according to research.

Individual preferences are influenced by a variety of factors, including heredity and personal experiences. Some people may have an inherent sensitivity to particular flavors or textures, making salads and vegetables less appealing to them.

Regardless of these issues, it is critical to include vegetables in our diet because they are high in nutrients, fiber, vitamins, and minerals, all of which contribute to general health. We may progressively modify our taste preferences and appreciate the benefits of veggies by being patient with ourselves and exploring different cooking methods, textures, and combinations.

The Science Of Taste Adjustment

Taste adaptation is a complex process influenced by several factors, including heredity, flavor exposure, and personal experiences. Our sense of taste changes and adapts to our surroundings, and our preferences vary as we get older. Taste receptors on the tongue play an important role in this process. Taste receptors are triggered when a person consumes food, and how we encode these tastes with meaning is a unique experience.

Exposure to different sensations shapes the evolving palette, and people learn to correlate tastes with outcomes. For example, after discovering that bitter tastes are not dangerous, someone may come to appreciate them, whereas bad experiences with particular meals can lead to aversion. This emphasizes the importance of learning and memory in taste adaptation.

Taste perception is also influenced by genetics. According to research, genes implicated in taste perception have not been positively selected in recent human evolution, implying that genetic differences among human groups regarding taste perception may exist. This genetic variation adds to variances in how people perceive and enjoy different tastes.

Furthermore, the human taste system evolved over millions of years in an environment dominated by food shortages. This evolutionary history has affected our perception of basic tastes like sweet, salty, sour, bitter, and umami, as well as extra attributes like fatty and metallic flavors.

Taste adaptation is a dynamic process that can be affected by repeated exposure to various flavors. Our taste buds can adjust and become more used to varied flavors over time by introducing a range of tastes into our diet and being open to exploring new foods. Consistency in exposing oneself to a variety of flavors is essential for building a liking for a wider range of foods.

Taste adaptation is a complex process that includes genetic, environmental, and experience components. Our perception of taste is not fixed and can change as a result of our exposure to diverse flavors and our own experiences. Individuals can extend their palate and gain a stronger appreciation for a diverse range of foods by learning the science behind taste adaptation.

The Advantages Of Eating Vegetables

Vegetables are an important part of a balanced diet since they provide several health advantages. They are high in nutrients such as vitamins, minerals, fiber, and antioxidants, which are essential for overall health and illness prevention. Among the many advantages of having vegetables in our diet are:

1. **Nutrient-dense:** Vegetables are high in nutrients like vitamin A, vitamin C, potassium, and folate. These nutrients are essential for a variety of body activities, including immunological function, eyesight, and the creation of red blood cells.

2. **Dietary Fiber:** Vegetables are high in dietary fiber, which is beneficial to digestive health and can help avoid constipation. Furthermore, fiber may aid in the absorption of vitamins and minerals in the body.

3. **Antioxidants:** Many veggies include antioxidants, including polyphenols and beta-carotene, which can help the body neutralize damaging free radicals. As a result, the risk of chronic diseases may be reduced, and healthy aging may be promoted.

4. **Low in Calories and Fats:** Because vegetables are low in calories and fats, they are an excellent choice for people trying to maintain a healthy weight. Their high nutrient

content also makes them an important part of a well-balanced diet.

5. **Disease Prevention:** Vegetable consumption is linked to a lower risk of a variety of chronic diseases, including heart disease, certain malignancies, and type 2 diabetes. Vegetables' broad array of nutrients and bioactive substances contribute to their beneficial effects.

Vegetables can be included in our meals in a variety of ways, including salads, soups, stews, or simply as a side dish. We can guarantee that we are obtaining a wide range of nutrients to support general health and well-being by having a variety of vegetables in our diet.

Vegetables are not only delicious and varied, but they also provide numerous health benefits. By making vegetables a regular component of our diet, we can improve our health, lower our risk of chronic diseases, and live a healthier and happier life.

Strategies For Enhancing The Flavor Of Salads And Vegetables

Salads and vegetables are key components of a balanced diet, but many individuals dislike them owing to their taste or texture. Fortunately, there are various methods for improving the flavor of salads and vegetables, making them more appealing to eat. Among these strategies are:

1. **Experiment with different preparations:** The way salads and vegetables are prepared can have a significant impact on their flavor and appeal. To bring out the natural sweetness and flavor of veggies, try roasting, grilling, or sautéing them. Experimenting with different textures, such as slicing veggies smaller or chunkier, can also aid in the discovery of a more appealing texture.

2. **Add flavor with seasonings and dressings:** Seasonings and dressings can help disguise the bitterness of vegetables and rapidly improve the taste of salads. Salad seasoning and dressing can help make salads taste nicer since salt and fat can diminish the impression of bitterness. Experiment with several dressings, such as vinaigrettes or creamy dressings, to find the one that best suits your palate.

3. **Experiment with different textures:** Salads are the ideal vehicle for a variety of textures, which can make your salad more intriguing and thus make you want to eat more of them. For a chewy texture, add dried fruit, nuts or seeds for crunch, and cottage cheese, goat cheese, or avocado for a creamy element. Changing your orange carrots for brilliant purple ones or adding a bag of multicolored cherry tomatoes can also bring diversity and interest to your salads.

4. **Include cooked vegetables:** Salad does not have to be all raw vegetables. Adding cooked vegetables to your salad is a terrific way to use up leftovers while also adding more nutrition. Salads can benefit from the addition of roasted veggies, grilled corn, or sautéed mushrooms.

5. **Pickling or fermenting:** Pickling or fermenting veggies can add zing to salads. Try quick pickled red onions or carrots with white vinegar and a little agave, then leave them for a few hours. Fermented vegetables, such as kimchi or sauerkraut, can also give a sour flavor to salads.

There are various methods for improving the flavor of salads and vegetables, making them more delightful to consume. Individuals can broaden their taste and gain a stronger appreciation for a diverse variety of foods by experimenting with different preparations, adding flavor with seasonings and sauces, mixing and matching components, including cooked vegetables, and pickling or fermenting.

Trying Out Different Textures And Combinations

Experimenting with different textures and combinations can greatly improve the appeal of salads and vegetables, making them more appealing to eat. Individuals can create intriguing and gratifying dining experiences by incorporating a range of textures and flavor combinations. The following are some useful ways to experiment with different textures and combinations:

1. **Use a range of textures:** Mixing textures such as crunchy, creamy, and chewy can add depth and intrigue to salads and vegetable meals. Adding nuts, seeds, or croutons to a salad, for example, can give it a pleasing crunch, while creamy additions like avocado or cheese can balance the texture.

2. **Balance flavors and mouth feels:**Pairing contrasting textures, such as crispy and tender or smooth and crunchy, can produce a more dynamic and delightful eating experience. A salad with crisp lettuce, creamy avocado, and crunchy veggies, for example, can provide a pleasant mixture of textures and flavors.

3. **Experiment with temperature:** Using items of varied temperatures, such as warm roasted vegetables over a bed of cool,

crisp greens, can lend dimension to the dish. The contrast between hot and cold components can add interest and satisfaction to the meal.

4. Experiment with complimentary ingredients: Combining sweet and savory flavors, for example, can improve the flavor of salads and vegetables. For example, adding fresh fruits to a salad, such as berries or citrus segments, can provide a nice burst of sweetness and acidity, boosting the overall flavor profile.

5. Experiment with global cuisines: Drawing inspiration from various culinary traditions can provide a variety of textures and taste combinations for salads and veggie meals. Incorporating components usually found in Asian, Mediterranean, or Latin American cuisines, for example, might bring new and fascinating flavor experiences.

Experimenting with different textures and combinations is a fun and effective method to improve the flavor and appearance of salads and vegetables. Individuals can create more dynamic, gratifying, and delightful dining experiences by incorporating a range of textures, balancing flavors and mouthfeels, playing with temperature, utilizing complementing ingredients, and studying world cuisines.

Putting Prejudices And Assumptions About Taste To The Test

Challenging our taste prejudices and assumptions is vital for widening our culinary horizons and enjoying the world's different cuisines. Genetics, cultural backgrounds, and personal experiences all have an impact on our taste preferences. We can become more receptive to experiencing new flavors and meals by questioning our assumptions and confronting our taste prejudices.

1. **Recognize and confront assumptions:** We all make assumptions about other people's likes based on demographics, cultural backgrounds, or personal preferences. It's is critical to challenge these preconceptions and be open to the notion that people's tastes differ greatly.

2. **Embrace the unusual:** It can be intimidating to try new flavors and foods, but it's critical to embrace the unfamiliar and approach food with an open mind. This allows us to discover new flavors and cuisines that we may appreciate.

3. **Cultural exchange:** Learning about diverse countries' culinary traditions might help us challenge our taste biases and broaden our palette. Experimenting with products and flavors from different cultures can introduce us to new and intriguing tasting experiences.

4. **Reevaluate taste choices:** Our taste preferences might alter as we mature and are exposed to new flavors. We can become more receptive to exploring new flavors by reevaluating our taste preferences and challenging our beliefs about what we like.

5. **Concentrate on the flavors we like:** Instead of focusing on the flavors we detest, focus on the flavors we like. We can teach our taste buds to be more open to a wider range of flavors by doing so.

Challenging taste prejudices and assumptions is vital for personal development and culinary inquiry. We can become more open to experiencing new flavors and foods by questioning our assumptions, accepting the unknown, engaging in cultural exchanges, reevaluating our taste preferences, and focusing on the flavors we enjoy. In turn, this can broaden our culinary experiences and contribute to a more diverse and satisfying diet.

Tips For Effective Taste Training

Various tactics and procedures can be used to produce successful taste training. Here are some pointers for effective taste training:

1. Introducing new flavors gradually: Introduce new flavors gradually to allow the palette to acclimate and become more sensitive to varied sensations. This can be accomplished through minor, incremental dietary modifications, such as introducing a new vegetable or fruit to meals.

2. Include a Variety of Meals: Eating a variety of meals will help teach the taste buds to appreciate varied flavors. Encouraging the consumption of foods with a variety of flavor characteristics, such as sweet, sour, bitter, and savory, can help to develop a more diverse and adaptive palette.

3. Hold Taste Tests and Tastings: Hold taste tests and tastings to encourage people to try new foods and flavors. This is especially good for children, as it makes eating new meals more pleasurable and less daunting.

4. Combine New Flavors with Familiar Dishes: Combining new or unpopular flavors with familiar or well-liked dishes might help make them more appealing. Incorporating a new vegetable into a favorite recipe or pairing it with a familiar ingredient or sauce, for example, can improve its appeal.

5. Be Mindful and Present During Meals: Promoting mindfulness during meals might help people pay more attention to the flavors and textures of the foods they eat. This can lead to a higher awareness of the sensory components of food and the development of a more refined palette.

A combination of gradual exposure to new sensations, incorporating a variety of foods, participating in taste tests and tastings, matching new flavors with familiar foods, and practicing awareness during meals is required for successful taste training. Individuals can broaden their palates and develop a stronger appreciation for a wide range of flavors and cuisines by applying these tactics.

Accepting The Taste Adaptation Journey

The journey of taste adaptation is an enthralling investigation of how our perception of taste changes and adapts to our surroundings. Genetics, cultural backgrounds, and personal experiences all have an impact on our taste preferences. We can become more receptive to exploring new flavors and cuisines if we embrace this journey, resulting in a more diverse and delightful culinary experience.

1. Genetic and Evolutionary Aspects: The human taste system evolved over millions of years as a result of food shortages. This evolutionary history has affected our perception of basic tastes like sweet, salty, sour, bitter, and umami, as well as extra attributes like fatty and metallic flavors. Recent research has also revealed that genes implicated in taste perception have not been positively selected in recent human evolution, implying that genetic differences between human groups may exist in terms of taste perception.

2. Cultural and Experiential Influences: Our cultural backgrounds and personal experiences shape our taste preferences. Exploring other cultural culinary traditions might help us challenge our taste biases and broaden our palette. Furthermore, reevaluating taste preferences and being willing to try new flavors might result in a more diverse and satisfying diet.

3. Taste Training and Adaptation: Taste adaptation is a dynamic process that can be altered by consistent flavor exposure. Exposure to new flavors gradually, integrating a range of foods, and participating in taste tests and tastings can all help train the taste buds to appreciate varied flavors. Individuals can broaden their palates and develop a stronger appreciation for a wide range of flavors and cuisines by applying these tactics.

Understanding the genetic and evolutionary components of taste perception, recognizing the influence of cultural and experiential influences on taste preferences, and actively engaging in taste training and adaptation are all part of the path of flavor adaptation. Individuals can expand their culinary experiences and create a more varied and adaptive palate by being open to experiencing new flavors, challenging taste prejudices, and exploring diverse culinary cultures.

Understanding Seasonal Vegetables

Understanding seasonal vegetables is vital for knowing what veggies are in season and when, and properly storing them can help guarantee that they stay fresh for as long as possible.

Seasonal vegetables are ones that are harvested and available at specific times of the year. Temperature and climatic factors influence the availability of seasonal vegetables. Seasonal veggies can be both globally and locally seasonal. Globally, seasonal vegetables are grown in their natural season and consumed anywhere in the world, whereas locally, seasonal vegetables are grown in their native season and consumed within the same climatic zone. Eating seasonal veggies provides various advantages, including enhanced nutrition, improved health and performance, and cost savings. Seasonal veggies are also good for the environment and the local economy. The availability of seasonal vegetables varies by region, so knowing what veggies are in season and when is vital. Seasonal veggies can be kept fresh for as long as possible by properly storing them. Most seasonal vegetables benefit from refrigeration, while others, such as onions, squash, pumpkin, turnips, and Swedish, benefit from storage in a cold, dark environment. Preparing and freezing veggies might also help increase their shelf life. A seasonal produce guide might assist you in discovering new fruits and vegetables throughout the year.

Oca Tubers: A Healthy Autumn Treat

Oca tubers are a nutrient-dense fall treat that can be consumed raw or cooked. They are an excellent source of carbs, vitamin C, iron, and potassium, as well as protein. Seasonal fruits and vegetables are accessible throughout the year, and eating locally seasonal food has numerous benefits for nutrition, the environment, the local economy, and even your bank account. A seasonal produce guide will help you discover new fruits and veggies all year long. Sheet pan chicken with vegetables is a quick, easy, and nutritious recipe ideal for busy weeknights. Keto-friendly vegetables are a low-carb joy that can be used to prepare salads, stir-fries, and soups. Weight Watchers vegetable soup is a hearty bowl of food that is ideal for a nutritious and substantial supper.

Recipes That Are Both Healthy And Delicious

Here are three healthy and delectable meals to try:

1. Weight Watchers Vegetable Soup: This soup is a hearty bowl of food that is ideal for a filling and healthy supper. The recipe can be found on Food.com or the Weight Watchers website. Nonfat vegetable or chicken broth, garlic, tomato paste, cabbage, onion, carrot, green beans, zucchini, basil, oregano, salt, and pepper are used to make this soup. It's a low-calorie, low-fat soup that's ideal for losing weight.

2. Sheet Pan Chicken and Veggies: Perfect for hectic weeknights, this meal is quick, easy, and healthy. The recipe may be found on All Day I Dream About Food [9]. Chicken thighs, cauliflower, Brussels sprouts, bacon, avocado oil, salt, pepper, butter, garlic, cumin, paprika, and coriander are used to make this recipe. It is a flavor-packed, low-carb, and keto-friendly recipe.

3. Keto-Friendly Vegetables: If you're searching for a low-carb treat, consider this Diet Doctor dish. A graphic guide to the best and worst keto vegetables is included in the recipe. Spinach, zucchini, lettuce, cucumbers, cabbage, asparagus, and kale are some of the greatest keto veggies. These low-carb vegetables are ideal for a keto diet. These vegetables can be used to produce a number of cuisines, including salads, stir-fries, and soups.

These meals are nutritious, tasty, and simple to prepare. They are ideal for anyone looking to eat healthily and maintain a balanced diet.

Making Nutritious Decisions

Understanding the different types of vegetables and their nutritional value can help you navigate healthy vegetable selections. Here are two different kinds of vegetables:

1. **Non-starchy veggies:** Low in carbohydrates, these veggies are suitable for those on a low-carb or ketogenic diet. Amaranth, or Chinese spinach; artichoke; asparagus; green beans; and cabbage are examples of non-starchy vegetables. Non-starchy veggies are high in vitamins, minerals, fiber, and phytochemicals, making them a nutritious addition to any diet.

2. **High-Protein Vegetables:** Protein, a crucial component for muscle growth and repair, is abundant in these vegetables. Spinach, Swiss chard, and beans are examples of high-protein vegetables. High-protein vegetables can be an important part of a well-balanced diet, particularly for vegetarians and vegans who need to ingest more plant-based proteins.

Understanding the many varieties of vegetables and their nutritional value will help you make healthier dietary choices. You can guarantee that you are getting a variety of critical nutrients by integrating a variety of veggies into your meals.

23

Vegetables For Weight Loss

When it comes to veggies for weight loss, including non-starchy vegetables in your diet might be really useful. Non-starchy veggies are low in calories and carbs, making them an ideal choice for weight loss and maintenance. Spinach, asparagus, broccoli, cauliflower, and bell peppers are examples of common non-starchy vegetables. These veggies are high in vitamins, minerals, and fiber and can be consumed in large quantities without negatively altering blood sugar levels. They can also be used to make a range of wonderful and filling meals, such as fresh vegetable soup and garden vegetable soup.

Furthermore, knowing the best veggies for low-carb and keto diets is critical for individuals trying to lose weight. Keto-friendly veggies like spinach, zucchini, lettuce, and cabbage are low in carbohydrates and can be consumed as part of a ketogenic diet. You may construct a balanced and nutritious diet that supports your weight loss objectives by integrating these vegetables into your meals.

Non-starchy vegetables and keto-friendly vegetables are beneficial to weight management. They contain necessary nutrients, contribute to a balanced diet, and can be utilized to make a variety of fulfilling and delicious recipes. You can efficiently manage your weight while enjoying a range of delectable and healthy meals if you include these vegetables in your diet.

Conclusion

We learn a lot as we grow and are exposed to diverse sensations, and we correlate distinct tastes with different outcomes. Taste receptors are meant to evolve and adapt to our surroundings, and our tastes vary as we get older. Understanding the genetic and evolutionary aspects of taste perception, recognizing the influence of cultural and experiential factors on taste preferences, and actively engaging in taste training and adaptation are all necessary for broadening our culinary horizons and embracing the world's diverse flavors. Individuals can expand their culinary experiences and create a more varied and adaptive palate by being open to experiencing new flavors, challenging taste prejudices, and exploring diverse culinary cultures.

www.ingramcontent.com/pod-product-compliance
Lightning Source LLC
Chambersburg PA
CBHW050757250726
48662CB00005B/2266